MATHA J. RUSSELL

BEYOND PICKY EATING

A Guide to Overcoming ARFID

Contents

INTRODUCTION

In our society, food is not just a source of nourishment but also an integral part of culture, social bonding, and comfort. However, people who have difficulty eating a variety of foods are often misunderstood or disregarded as being "picky eaters." In reality, this seemingly harmless term masks a complex and debilitating disorder called Avoidant/Restrictive Food Intake Disorder (ARFID).

Think about a child who refuses to eat anything other than a few specific meals or an adult who is afraid to try new foods and feels frustrated by the limited options available to them. These are not just preferences or whims; they are signs of a deep-rooted struggle with food that goes beyond the dinner table.

But there is hope. This book aims to help readers understand the nuances of selective eating and uncover the mystery of ARFID with compassion and competence. We will explore the roots and impact of this disorder, and most importantly, how to overcome it. This book is more than just a collection of pages; it is a lifeline for those experiencing ARFID and a source of hope for their loved ones.

I

Part 1 : Understanding ARFID

1

Chapter One

What is ARFID?

I n a world where food is abundant and varied, it's tempting to believe that everyone eats a varied and balanced meal. However, for people suffering from Avoidant/Restrictive Food Intake Disorder (ARFID), even eating can be difficult and stressful.

Unraveling the Complexity of ARFID

Imagine sitting down to eat, only to be overcome with terror and dread at the sight of unknown cuisine. This is the reality for people who have ARFID, a syndrome marked by a strong dislike for specific foods, textures, colors, or odors. Unlike fussy eaters, who may just have strong preferences, people with ARFID suffer true difficulty and discomfort when exposed to new or unfamiliar foods.

Symptoms of ARFID

ARFID symptoms might vary greatly from person to person, however, some typical markers are:

1. **Severe dietary restriction:** People with ARFID frequently have a very limited selection of foods that they will eat, resulting in nutritional deficits and poor health effects.
2. **Fear or anxiety over food:** Even the prospect of trying new foods can cause acute anxiety or panic episodes in those with ARFID.
3. **Sensory sensitivities:** Many patients with ARFID have hypersensitive sensory systems, making particular textures, odors, and tastes unbearable.
4. **Avoidance of social situations involving food:** Because of their restricted diet, people with ARFID may avoid social events or eating out with friends and family, causing feelings of isolation and loneliness.

Diagnosing ARFID

Diagnosing ARFID can be difficult because it frequently coexists with other mental health illnesses like anxiety disorders or autism spectrum disorder. Healthcare practitioners usually seek the following criteria when making a diagnosis:

- Persistent food avoidance or restriction results in severe weight loss or failure to meet nutritional needs.
- Significant disruption to social, occupational, or other critical areas of functioning.
- ARFID differs from other eating disorders such as anorexia nervosa and bulimia nervosa in that there is no alteration in body image or fear of gaining weight.

Distinguishing ARFID from Picky Eating

While picky eating and ARFID have certain similarities, there are major characteristics that distinguish them:

- **Severity:** Picky eating is characterized by minor preferences or dislikes for specific foods, but ARFID is characterized by severe aversions that have a major impact on everyday life and functioning.
- **Distress:**Picky eaters may feel hesitant or uncomfortable when eating new foods, but people with ARFID experience intense dread and anxiety.
- **Nutritional consequences:** Despite their preferences, picky eaters can maintain a balanced diet, but people with ARFID are at risk of nutritional deficits and other health issues due to their restricted consumption.

2

Chapter Two

Understanding the Roots of ARFID

I magine sitting down to a meal only to be paralyzed by anxiety and discomfort at the prospect of attempting anything outside your small repertoire of safe meals. For people suffering from Avoidant/Restrictive Food Intake Disorder (ARFID), this predicament is a daily reality rather than a hypothetical one. This chapter investigates the numerous foundations of ARFID, which include biological, sensory, emotional, and developmental components.

Biological factors

At the heart of ARFID are complex biochemical factors that influence a person's relationship with food. Research reveals that genetic predispositions may influence food choices and aversions. Furthermore, neurobiological variations in brain structure and function can lead to increased sensory sensitivities, rendering particular foods unpalatable to those with ARFID. For example, people with ARFID may have heightened gag reflexes or sensory processing difficulties that make it difficult to accept particular textures or flavors.

Sensory factors

Our eating habits and preferences are heavily influenced by our sensory experiences with food. Sensory sensitivities can be overpowering for people with ARFID, causing them to avoid certain textures, odors, and tastes. For example, the texture of some foods may cause pain or even revulsion, making it hard for those with ARFID to eat them. Understanding these sensory sensitivities is critical to creating effective interventions and accommodations for people with ARFID.

Emotional Factors

Food is more than just a source of nutrition; it is also intimately linked to our emotions and social experiences. Emotional elements like worry, fear, or trauma can have a substantial impact on a person's connection with food and contribute to the development of ARFID. An unpleasant event with food, such as choking or food poisoning, may result in a long-term aversion to certain foods or textures. Similarly, people with anxiety disorders may have increased worry over food, making it difficult for them to try new cuisines or eat in unfamiliar settings.

Developmental Factors

The early years of development are essential for forming our attitudes and behaviors towards eating. Children who have eating issues or disturbances in early childhood may be more likely to develop ARFID later in adulthood. For example, infants who struggle with breastfeeding or transitioning to solid foods may develop aversions to specific textures or flavors. Similarly, children who have bad mealtime relationships or are pressured to eat may develop anxiety or aversions to food, laying the groundwork for ARFID to emerge.

Integrating the factors

While each of these factors biological, sensory, emotional, and developmental plays a unique role in creating ARFID, it is critical to understand how they are interrelated and influence one another in complicated ways. For example, a biological predisposition to heightened sensory sensitivity may mix with emotional factors such as anxiety or trauma to aggravate food aversions. Similarly, developmental variables such as early feeding challenges may contribute to the development of ARFID by molding an individual's beliefs and behaviors around food.

3

Chapter Three

The Impact of ARFID

Aside from the surface-level issues of avoiding certain foods, people with Avoidant/Restrictive Food Intake Disorder (ARFID) encounter a complicated web of challenges every day. This chapter explores how ARFID affects physical health, mental well-being, and social life, giving light to the complex nature of this often misunderstood condition.

Physical Toll

At its heart, ARFID poses major physical health hazards due to severe food restrictions and resulting nutritional deficits. Individuals with ARFID frequently have a narrow range of safe foods that they are willing to ingest, resulting in nutritional imbalances such as vitamins, minerals, and macronutrients. As a result, individuals may face a variety of physical health issues, such as:

- **Malnutrition:** The restrictive nature of ARFID can result in insufficient calorie and vital nutrient intake, leading to malnutrition and its related health effects.
- **Weight loss or failure to thrive:** Children with ARFID may have difficulty

gaining weight and growing normally, resulting in developmental delays and growth stunting.

- **Gastrointestinal issues:**ARFID can aggravate gastrointestinal disorders like constipation, bloating, and abdominal pain, aggravating the eating experience.
- **Weak immune system:** Nutritional inadequacies caused by ARFID can impair the immune system, making people more vulnerable to infections and diseases.

Mental Strain

Aside from the physical toll, ARFID has a substantial influence on people's emotional and psychological health. The widespread anxiety and dread of food can contribute to a variety of mental health concerns, including:

- **Anxiety disorders:** Many people with ARFID have high levels of anxiety around eating, which can lead to panic attacks, phobias, and other anxiety-related symptoms.
- **Depression:** The chronic stress and isolation associated with ARFID can exacerbate feelings of sadness, hopelessness, and despair, leading to depression in some cases.
- **Low self-esteem:** Living with ARFID can damage people's confidence and self-worth, resulting in poor self-perceptions and low self-esteem.
- **Body image issues:** While ARFID is not motivated by concerns about weight or shape, individuals may develop skewed body image beliefs as a result of their restrictive eating habits.

Social Isolation

ARFID has an impact not only on people's physical and mental health, but also on their social lives, disrupting relationships, social interactions, and a sense of belonging. Individuals with ARFID may experience social isolation and withdrawal as a result of their pervasive anxiety and dread of food. Some common social issues faced by individuals with ARFID are:

- **Difficulty eating out:** People with ARFID may struggle to find safe meals when dining out, causing anxiety and discomfort in social situations like restaurants or gatherings.
- **Feeling misunderstood:** Friends, family members, and even healthcare experts frequently misunderstand ARFID, leading to feelings of isolation and alienation for those suffering from the illness.
- **Relationship impact:** ARFID can affect relationships with friends and family members who do not understand or support the individual's dietary limitations, resulting in conflict and tension.
- **Limited social activities:** Fear and anxiety over eating can cause people with ARFID to avoid social activities involving food, adding to feelings of isolation and loneliness.

II

Part 2 : A Guide to Overcoming ARFID

4

Chapter Four

Creating Your Support Network

Navigating the hurdles of Avoidant/Restrictive Food Intake Disorder (ARFID) can be difficult, but you don't have to do it alone. This chapter discusses the significance of establishing a solid support network to assist you on your path to recovery. From therapists and nutritionists to the steadfast support of family and friends, leveraging your support network can make all the difference in overcoming ARFID.

The Role of Therapists

Therapists play an important role in the treatment of ARFID by giving people the tools and methods they need to overcome their obstacles and create a healthier connection with their food. Cognitive Behavioural Therapy (CBT), in particular, has been demonstrated to be useful in treating ARFID by assisting clients in identifying and challenging negative food-related thoughts and beliefs. Individual therapy sessions allow therapists to work with clients to address the underlying psychological causes that contribute to their ARFID and develop coping mechanisms to manage their anxiety and fear of eating.

Nutritionists

Nutritionists are critical members of the ARFID support team, providing individuals with practical advice and help to ensure they satisfy their nutritional requirements despite their restricted diets. Nutritionists may assist individuals in identifying safe foods that contain the key nutrients they require to flourish, as well as developing meal plans and dietary strategies to ensure they are eating a balanced and diverse diet. Individuals with ARFID who work closely with nutritionists can learn to make smart diet choices and overcome their anxiety about eating new foods.

The Power of Family and Friendship

Individuals with ARFID may find that their family and friends are the most valuable sources of support. The constant love, compassion, and encouragement of loved ones can provide individuals with the strength and drive they require to persevere on their path to recovery. Family and friends can actively support individuals with ARFID by:

- **Creating a supportive meal environment:** Family members can provide a secure and friendly meal atmosphere that is free of pressure or judgement, allowing people with ARFID to eat at their own pace and comfort level.
- **Encouraging exposure to new foods:** Loving ones can gently urge people with ARFID to try new foods in a caring and non-coercive manner, appreciating each small step forward.
- **Providing emotional support:** ARFID may be emotionally difficult, so having a solid support system in place can make all the difference. Family members and friends can provide a listening ear, words of encouragement, and unconditional love to assist individuals in navigating the ups and downs of their recovery process.

5

Chapter Five

Cultivating Self-Compassion and Acceptance

One of the most transforming aspects of resolving Avoidant/Restrictive Food Intake Disorder (ARFID) is to cultivate self-compassion and acceptance. In this chapter we go on a journey to understand the triggers and feelings that come with ARFID, as well as how practicing self-compassion can lead to healing and progress.

Understanding Triggers

Triggers are the catalysts that cause people with ARFID to feel anxious, fearful, or uncomfortable around food. These triggers can vary greatly from person to person, but some popular examples are:

- **Texture:** specific textures of food can cause discomfort or even disgust in people with ARFID, making it difficult for them to eat specific meals.
- **Smell:** In people with ARFID, strong or unexpected smells can cause anxiety and aversion, making it difficult for them to try new foods or eat in unfamiliar settings.
- **Appearance:** The appearance of specific foods, such as their color or shape,

can cause anxiety or dread in people with ARFID, leading to avoidance or limitation of certain items.

- **Past Trauma:** Traumatic experiences with food, such as choking or food poisoning, can be potent triggers for people with ARFID, resulting in long-term aversions or concerns about certain meals.

Individuals with ARFID can begin to build skills for controlling their anxiety and discomfort around food by identifying and understanding their triggers, allowing them to eventually take control of their eating behaviors and choices.

Navigating Emotions

ARFID rehabilitation is loaded with complicated feelings, including dread, worry, frustration, and self-doubt. Individuals with ARFID should recognize and affirm their feelings, rather than ignoring or repressing them. Some prevalent emotions reported by individuals with ARFID are:

- **Fear:** Fear is a ubiquitous emotion for people with ARFID, resulting from their worry and discomfort around eating. Fear of choking, vomiting, and trying new foods are all prominent signs of ARFID-related anxiety.
- **Frustration:** Frustration is a natural reaction to the challenges and disappointments encountered on the path to ARFID recovery. Individuals with ARFID may experience dissatisfaction at various stages of their recovery process, ranging from difficulty finding safe foods to feeling misunderstood.
- **Shame:** Shame is a particularly pernicious feeling for people with ARFID, who may feel guilty or embarrassed about their eating habits and preferences. Overcoming feelings of shame and self-judgment is critical to developing self-compassion and acceptance.
- **Hope:** Despite the hardships of ARFID, many people discover hope and perseverance on their path to recovery. Individuals with ARFID can foster a sense of hope and optimism about the future by focusing on modest successes and progress.

Cultivating Self-Compassion

Self compassion is the discipline of treating oneself with kindness, understanding, and acceptance, particularly in the face of difficulties or disappointments. For people with ARFID, fostering self-compassion is critical for managing the complexity of their disease with grace and perseverance. Here are some techniques to build self-compassion:

- **Practice mindfulness:** Mindfulness is the practice of bringing awareness to the current moment without passing judgment. Individuals with ARFID can improve their self-awareness and acceptance by practicing mindfulness.
- **Challenge negative self-talk:** Negative self-talk can prevent self-compassion by reinforcing feelings of shame and self-judgment. Individuals with ARFID can create a more sympathetic inner dialogue by challenging their negative self-talk and replacing it with positive affirmations.
- **Seek support:** Creating a solid support network of friends, family, and healthcare professionals is critical for developing self-compassion and acceptance. Surrounding oneself with sympathetic and understanding people can provide a sense of affirmation and encouragement on the path to ARFID recovery.
- **Practice self-care:** Self-care is the practice of putting one's physical, emotional, and mental well-being first. Individuals with ARFID can develop a stronger feeling of self-compassion and acceptance by participating in activities that nourish and renew the body and mind.

Embracing Acceptance

Acceptance is the willingness to recognize and appreciate one's ideas, feelings, and experiences without judgment or resistance. For those with ARFID, acceptance is admitting their dietary challenges and understanding that recovery is a journey, not a destination. Acceptance allows people with ARFID to create a sense of calm and empowerment in their connection with food and themselves.

6

Chapter Six

Creating a Safe and Predictable Meal Environment

This chapter discusses the necessity of having a safe and predictable meal environment for people dealing with Avoidant/Restrictive Food Intake Disorder (ARFID). Understanding sensory considerations and applying appropriate meal planning tactics can help people with ARFID approach mealtimes with confidence and ease, opening the path for a healthier relationship with food.

Understanding Sensory Considerations

Individuals with ARFID rely heavily on their sensory experiences with food to determine their eating habits and preferences. specific textures, scents, colors, and tastes might cause discomfort, anxiety, or even revulsion, making it difficult for people with ARFID to eat specific meals. As a result, it's critical to consider sensory characteristics while designing a meal environment for people with ARFID. Some sensory considerations to keep in mind are:

- **Texture:** Texture is one of the most important sensory aspects for people with ARFID. Certain textures, such as mushy or slimy textures, may cause pain or gagging in people with ARFID. As a result, providing a variety of textures and allowing people with ARFID to select foods that feel comfortable to them can help reduce their anxiety about mealtimes.

- **Smell:** Strong or new smells can cause anxiety and aversion in people with ARFID. As a result, it is critical to avoid overwhelming fragrances in the meal area and offer appropriate ventilation to reduce strong odors.
- **Visual Presentation:** The appearance of food can also influence those with ARFID. Certain colors or forms may cause anxiety or discomfort, prompting people to avoid or restrict certain foods. As a result, presenting foods in a visually appealing manner and providing a variety of colors and forms might help make mealtimes more inviting for those with ARFID.
- **Temperature:** The temperature of food can also impact people with ARFID. Some people prefer meals at room temperature, while others prefer it hot or cold. As a result, while arranging meals for people with ARFID, it is critical to consider their preferred temperature.

By recognizing and respecting sensory issues, we may create a meal atmosphere that is safe, comfortable, and inviting for people with ARFID, allowing them to try new foods and extend their nutritional repertoire.

Effective meal planning strategies

Meal planning is a vital part of providing a safe and predictable meal setting for people with ARFID. By carefully planning and preparing meals ahead of time, we may help ease anxiety and uncertainty about mealtimes and ensure that people with ARFID have access to foods that feel safe and familiar to them. Some helpful meal-planning options for people with ARFID are:

- **Establishing a schedule:** Having a consistent mealtime schedule might make people with ARFID feel more confident and in control of their eating environment. Set regular mealtimes and adhere to them as much as possible to provide structure and predictability to your day.
- **Offering Choices:** Giving people with ARFID a sense of autonomy and

control over their food choices can help them discover new foods at their own pace. Provide a variety of options and allow people to choose foods that they feel secure and familiar with.

- **Gradual Exposure:** Gradual exposure to novel foods is essential for helping people with ARFID increase their dietary range. Introduce new meals cautiously and gradually, beginning with small amounts and increasing exposure over time. Be patient and supportive, and applaud every small step forward.

- **Creating a Positive Meal Setting:** Create a welcoming and supportive mealtime setting free of pressure and judgement. Encourage open discussion and establish an atmosphere of acceptance and understanding at the table. Celebrate victories and milestones, no matter how little, and offer encouragement and support to those with ARFID as they work towards recovery.

7

Chapter Seven

Relaxation Techniques for Managing Anxiety Around Food

Chapter 7 discusses the relevance of relaxation strategies for reducing food-related anxiety. Mealtimes for people suffering from Avoidant/Restrictive Food Intake Disorder (ARFID) can be stressful, frightening, and uncomfortable. Individuals with ARFID who incorporate relaxation techniques into their daily routine can build a sense of peace and ease, allowing them to approach food with confidence and resilience.

Understanding Anxiety About Food

Individuals with ARFID frequently experience food anxiety, which can be attributed to a range of variables such as sensory sensitivity, fear of choking or vomiting, and previous traumatic events. This worry can show as bodily symptoms such as a racing heart, sweating, trembling, or nausea, making it difficult for those with ARFID to eat comfortably or try new foods. As a result, it is critical to create effective ways to reduce food anxiety and encourage calm during mealtimes.

Relaxation techniques

Deep breathing exercises are a simple but effective approach to relax and reduce anxiety. Encourage people with ARFID to practise deep breathing exercises before and during meals to help them relax and reduce their anxiety. Diaphragmatic breathing is an efficient deep breathing method in which people inhale deeply through their nose, allowing their abdomen to expand, and then gently exhale through their mouth, relieving tension and stress with each breath.

Progressive Muscle Relaxation (PMR)

Progressive Muscle Relaxation (PMR) is a stress-reduction technique that involves gradually tensing and releasing various muscle groups in the body. Encourage people with ARFID to use PMR before meals to relieve tension and anxiety. Begin by tensing and relaxing the muscles in your feet, then work your way up the body, concentrating on each muscle group and allowing it to fully relax before moving on to the next.

Visualization and Guided Imagery

Visualization and guided imagery are effective relaxing techniques that use mental images or scenarios to relieve anxiety. Encourage people with ARFID to imagine themselves in a quiet and calming setting, such as a tranquil beach or a serene forest. Guided imagery scripts can also be beneficial since they guide people through a succession of soothing scenes and encourage them to use their senses to induce relaxation.

Mindfulness Meditation

Mindfulness meditation is a technique that focuses on the present moment without judgment, promoting calmness and acceptance. Encourage people with ARFID to practise mindfulness meditation before meals to help them relax and reduce their anxiety. Simple mindfulness techniques like mindful breathing and body scan meditation can help promote relaxation and reduce stress.

Grounding Techniques

Grounding practices assist individuals stay connected to the present moment, minimizing anxiety and overload. Encourage people with ARFID to practise grounding techniques before meals to help them relax and reduce their anxiety. Simple grounding practices, such as focusing on the sensations of their feet on the ground or counting the objects in the room, can help people feel more grounded and centered, lowering anxiety and stress.

8

Chapter Eight

Cognitive Behavioral Therapy (CBT) for ARFID

This Chapter looks at how Cognitive Behavioural Therapy (CBT) can help treat Avoidant/Restrictive Food Intake Disorder (ARFID). As people with ARFID manage the complexities of their connection with food, addressing negative ideas and beliefs is critical for developing growth, resilience, and, eventually, recovery. Individuals with ARFID can use CBT to identify and address harmful cognitive patterns, opening the path for a healthier and more balanced relationship with food.

Understanding Cognitive-Behavioral Therapy (CBT)

Cognitive Behavioural Therapy (CBT) is an organized, goal-oriented type of psychotherapy that aims to identify and change problematic thought patterns and behaviors. In the setting of ARFID, CBT attempts to assist individuals in challenging their mistaken ideas and attitudes about food, ultimately encouraging them to create healthier eating habits and attitudes. CBT for ARFID typically consists of several critical components, including:

- **Psychoeducation:** Informing people with ARFID on the nature of their disorder, including symptoms, causes, and treatment choices. Psychoeducation assists individuals in better understanding their condition and promotes a sense of empowerment and control over their treatment process.

- **Cognitive Restructuring:** Assisting individuals in identifying and challenging negative food-related ideas and beliefs. Cognitive restructuring entails challenging the validity of negative ideas, uncovering evidence to support more balanced and realistic beliefs, and adopting new, more adaptive ways of thinking about food and eating.

- **Exposure Therapy:** Exposure Therapy is the gradual exposure of people with ARFID to foods they fear or avoid in a controlled and supportive environment. Exposure therapy assists individuals in confronting their concerns and worries about food, allowing them to gradually expand their nutritional repertoire and build greater flexibility and confidence in their eating behaviors.

- **Behavioral Experiments:** Through controlled behavioral experiments, people are encouraged to try out new food-related behaviors and attitudes. Behavioral studies enable people to question their assumptions and beliefs about food and eating, offering actual data to support more adaptive and healthy eating habits.

- **Skill Development:** Teaching people with ARFID practical skills and strategies for coping with anxiety, managing stress, and regulating their emotions around food and eating. Relaxation techniques, mindfulness practices, and problem-solving tactics can all be used to help people navigate difficult situations and stay on track with their recovery.

Challenging Negative Thoughts and Beliefs

Negative ideas and beliefs about food are common in people with ARFID, resulting in emotions of fear, anxiety, and avoidance around mealtimes. Individuals with ARFID can use CBT to identify and confront negative cognitive patterns, resulting in improved resilience and flexibility in their relationship with food. Some frequent negative views and perceptions about ARFID include:

- **All-or-nothing thinking:** Individuals with ARFID may exhibit all-or-nothing thinking, categorizing items as "safe" or "unsafe" and avoiding anything outside of their narrow spectrum of safe foods. This black-and-white thinking can exacerbate emotions of anxiety and avoidance around food, making it difficult for people to try new foods or broaden their dietary options.

- **Catastrophizing:** Catastrophizing refers to exaggerating the anticipated negative repercussions of trying new meals or eating outside of one's comfort zone. Individuals with ARFID may overestimate the likelihood of choking, vomiting or experiencing significant discomfort while sampling new foods.

- **Self-criticism:** People with ARFID may have self-critical thoughts and attitudes about their eating habits, perceiving themselves as weak, insufficient, or abnormal for facing food-related issues. This self-criticism can lower self-esteem and confidence, reinforcing bad eating habits and attitudes.

- **Perfectionism:** Perfectionism entails creating unnecessarily high expectations for oneself and feeling enormous pressure to reach these standards. Individuals with ARFID may feel pressured to eat "perfectly" or follow strict dietary rules and routines, which can lead to emotions of anger, guilt, and humiliation when they fall short of these expectations.

- **Avoidance:** Avoidance is the active avoidance of situations, foods, or activities that make you feel anxious or uncomfortable. Individuals with ARFID may engage in avoidance behaviors to cope with their food-related anxiety, reinforcing negative thoughts and prolonging the cycle of avoidance and worry.

Individuals with ARFID can begin to create a more balanced and realistic view of food and eating by identifying and confronting these negative ideas and beliefs through cognitive behavioral therapy, ultimately allowing them to overcome their worries and anxiety about mealtimes.

Practical Strategies for Combating Negative Thoughts and Beliefs

- **Thought logs:** Encourage people with ARFID to keep track of their negative ideas and attitudes about food using thought logs. Thought logs assist individuals in seeing patterns in their thinking and challenging the veracity of negative attitudes, resulting in more balanced and realistic approaches to food and eating.

- **Cognitive Restructuring:** Teach people with ARFID how to use cognitive restructuring tools to counter harmful thoughts and beliefs. Encourage them to seek out data that both supports and contradicts their negative ideas, as well as to create more adaptive and realistic attitudes towards food and eating.

- **Behavioral Experiments:** Encourage people with ARFID to try out new food-related behaviors and beliefs through controlled behavioral experiments. Allow individuals to gradually expose themselves to feared or avoided foods in a safe and supportive atmosphere, allowing them to confront their fears and anxieties while gathering evidence to challenge their negative views.

- **Graded Exposure:** Using a graded exposure technique, gradually expose people with ARFID to foods they fear or avoid. Begin with less anxiety-provoking meals and gradually increase exposure over time, allowing people to gain confidence and tolerance for new cuisines at their own pace.

- **Self-Compassion:** Encourage people with ARFID to be compassionate and kind to themselves as they navigate their recovery journey. Remind them that it is acceptable to struggle and make mistakes and that growth is not always linear. Encourage them to foster patience, understanding, and self-acceptance as they seek to overcome their food and eating difficulties.

9

Chapter Nine

Exposure Therapy for ARFID

In this chapter, we embark on a transformative journey of Exposure Therapy, a cornerstone of treatment for Avoidant/Restrictive Food Intake Disorder (ARFID). Exposure Therapy offers individuals with ARFID a structured and supportive framework for gradually introducing new foods into their diet, empowering them to confront their fears and anxieties surrounding food with courage and resilience. Through the process of systematic exposure, individuals with ARFID can expand their dietary repertoire, overcome their avoidance behaviors, and ultimately reclaim their relationship with food.

Understanding Exposure Therapy

Exposure Therapy is a well-established behavioral intervention that involves gradually exposing individuals to feared or avoided stimuli in a controlled and supportive environment. In the context of ARFID, Exposure Therapy aims to help individuals confront their fears and anxieties surrounding food by gradually introducing them to new and challenging foods in a systematic and structured manner. Exposure Therapy for ARFID typically involves several key components, including:

1. **Hierarchy Development:** Collaboratively developing a hierarchy of feared or avoided foods based on their level of anxiety or discomfort. The hierarchy allows individuals with ARFID to prioritize which foods they are ready to confront first and provides a roadmap for gradually increasing exposure over time.

2. **Exposure Planning:** Creating exposure plans that outline specific goals, strategies, and timelines for introducing new foods into individuals' diets. Exposure plans are tailored to each individual's unique needs and preferences, taking into account their level of readiness, past experiences, and areas of challenge

3. **Gradual Exposure:** Gradually exposing individuals to feared or avoided foods using a step-by-step approach. Exposure typically begins with foods that are less anxiety-provoking and gradually progresses to more challenging foods as individuals build confidence and tolerance over time.

4. **Coping Strategies:** Teaching individuals coping strategies and relaxation techniques to help them manage anxiety and discomfort during exposure exercises. Coping strategies may include deep breathing exercises, progressive muscle relaxation, and positive self-talk to help individuals stay calm and focused during exposure sessions. Support and

5. **Feedback:** Providing ongoing support and feedback throughout the exposure process to help individuals navigate their fears and challenges with food. Supportive encouragement and positive reinforcement can help individuals feel empowered and motivated to continue their progress in exposure therapy.

The Role of Exposure Therapy in ARFID Recovery

Exposure Therapy plays a crucial role in the treatment of ARFID, offering individuals a structured and supportive framework for confronting their fears and anxieties surrounding food. By systematically exposing individuals to feared or avoided foods, Exposure Therapy helps individuals build confidence, tolerance, and flexibility in their eating behaviors, ultimately empowering them to expand their dietary repertoire and overcome their avoidance behaviors. Some key benefits of Exposure Therapy for ARFID recovery include:

- **Increased Food Tolerance:** Exposure Therapy helps individuals gradually build tolerance to new and challenging foods, reducing feelings of anxiety and discomfort surrounding mealtimes.
- **Expanded Dietary Repertoire:** By systematically introducing new foods into individuals' diets, Exposure Therapy helps individuals expand their dietary repertoire and develop a more varied and balanced diet.
- **Improved Eating Behaviors:** Exposure Therapy helps individuals develop healthier eating behaviors and attitudes by challenging avoidance behaviors and fostering a more positive relationship with food. Enhanced **Quality of Life:** By overcoming their fears and anxieties surrounding food, individuals with ARFID can enjoy a greater sense of freedom, flexibility, and enjoyment in their eating experiences, ultimately leading to an improved quality of life.

Practical Strategies for Implementing Exposure Therapy

1. **Create a Fear Hierarchy:** Collaboratively develop a hierarchy of feared or avoided foods with the individual, starting with foods that evoke mild anxiety or discomfort and gradually progressing to more challenging foods.
2. **Set Realistic Goals:** Set achievable goals for exposure sessions, taking into account the individual's level of readiness, past experiences, and areas of challenge. Start with small, manageable steps and gradually increase the difficulty of exposure exercises over time.
3. **Provide Support and Encouragement:** Offer ongoing support and encouragement throughout the exposure process, acknowledging the individual's bravery and progress in confronting their fears and anxieties surrounding food. Practice Relaxation

4. **Techniques:** Teach individuals relaxation techniques and coping strategies to help them manage anxiety and discomfort during exposure exercises. Encourage individuals to practice deep breathing, progressive muscle relaxation, and positive self-talk to stay calm and focused during exposure sessions.

5. **Monitor Progress:** Regularly monitor progress and adjust exposure plans as needed based on the individual's feedback and experiences. Celebrate successes and milestones along the way, no matter how small, and provide positive reinforcement to help individuals stay motivated and engaged in the exposure process.

III

Part 3 : Expanding Your Diet and Living Well with ARFID

10

Chapter Ten

Nutritional Considerations for ARFID

Chapter 10 goes into the critical topic of nutritional considerations for those with Avoidant/Restrictive Food Intake Disorder (ARFID). While ARFID brings distinct obstacles in terms of food intake and diversity, maintaining a balanced and nourishing diet is critical for general health and well-being. Understanding the nutritional needs of people with ARFID and applying techniques to ensure balanced consumption of safe foods will help them thrive on their road to recovery.

Understanding ARFID and Nutritional Challenges

ARFID is distinguished by very selective eating behaviors, limited food intake, and avoidance of specific foods or food groups due to sensory sensitivity, fear of negative consequences, or other psychological causes. As a result, people with ARFID frequently suffer nutritional issues that affect their physical health, growth, and development. Some common nutritional difficulties related to ARFID are:

- **Limited Food Diversity:** People with ARFID may have a limited range of safe foods that they feel comfortable consuming, resulting in a limited dietary diversity and potential nutritional deficiencies.

- **Imbalanced Nutrient Intake:** Because of their limited food options, people with ARFID may struggle to get all of the nutrients their bodies require for good health and function. This can lead to an imbalance in nutrient intake and deficiencies in essential vitamins, minerals, and macronutrients.
- **Difficulty Meeting Energy Needs:** People with ARFID may struggle to eat enough calories to meet their energy requirements, particularly if they avoid calorie-dense or high-fat meals. This can result in low energy intake, weight loss, and weariness.
- **Malnutrition Risk:** Prolonged restrictions on specific foods or food groups might raise the risk of malnutrition in people with ARFID, compromising their physical health, growth, and development over time.
- **Impact on Mental Health:** ARFID-related nutritional problems can have a substantial impact on people's mental health and well-being, contributing to feelings of anxiety, despair, and low self-esteem.

Nutritional Considerations for ARFID Recovery:

Despite the obstacles provided by ARFID, it is feasible to assist individuals in reaching a balanced and nourishing diet by focusing on nutritional concerns that are specific to their requirements and tastes. Some important concerns for assisting individuals with ARFID in obtaining a balanced intake of safe foods include:

- **Identify Safe and Preferred Foods:** Collaborate with ARFID users to identify their safe and preferred foods, as well as any foods or food groups they are willing to add to their diet. Understanding people's dietary preferences and aversions is critical for creating a personalized nutrition plan that fits their nutritional demands while also respecting their comfort level with food.
- **Emphasise Nutrient-Dense Foods:** Encourage people with ARFID to consume nutrient-dense meals that include critical vitamins, minerals,

and macronutrients in tiny quantities. Nutrient-dense foods such as fruits, vegetables, lean meats, whole grains, and healthy fats can help people satisfy their nutritional needs without overeating.

- **Incorporate variation Within Safe meals:** While persons with ARFID may have a restricted selection of safe meals, it is critical to encourage variation within those foods to ensure a balanced nutritional intake. For example, if a person prefers chicken nuggets as a safe protein source, experiment with different cooking methods (e.g., baked, grilled) and seasoning combinations to give variety to their diet.

- **Offer Fortified Foods and Supplements:** If persons with ARFID are unable to receive adequate nutrients from food alone, try providing fortified foods or supplements to cover nutritional gaps. Fortified foods, such as fortified cereals, plant-based milk replacements, and meal replacement shakes, can deliver extra vitamins and minerals, whereas supplements, such as multivitamins or omega-3 fatty acids, can improve overall health and well-being.

- **Provide Supportive Meal Environment:** Create a meal atmosphere that encourages relaxation, comfort, and good food associations for people with ARFID. Reduce distractions, provide encouragement and appreciation, and avoid pressing people to eat foods they dislike. Individuals with ARFID might feel calmer and at ease during mealtimes by creating a safe and supportive meal setting, making it simpler for them to experiment with new foods and broaden their dietary repertoire.

Strategies for Ensuring Balanced Intake of Safe Foods:

- **Meal Planning and Preparation:** Collaborate with persons with ARFID to create meal plans that include a variety of safe foods and promote balanced nutrition. To provide a varied range of nutrients, include foods from many food groups (for example, fruits, vegetables, proteins, and grains). Involve people in meal planning and preparation activities to boost their engagement and ownership of their nutritional decisions.

- **Gradual introduction to new foods:** Gradual exposure approaches can help people with ARFID become more comfortable sampling new foods. Begin by introducing small amounts of new foods alongside known and preferred meals, gradually increasing exposure over time as people become more open to trying new flavors and textures.

- **Texture Modification:** Experiment with varied textures and preparations of safe foods to provide diversity in people's diets. Pureeing vegetables into soups or sauces, combining fruits into smoothies, and baking foods to generate varied textures can all help make them more edible and enticing to people with ARFID.

- **Encourage Self-Monitoring:** Individuals with ARFID should keep a food diary or journal to document their food intake and nutritional status. This can help people become more conscious of their eating patterns and identify areas for improvement, as well as give useful information for healthcare experts to monitor progress and provide nutritional recommendations.

- **Seek professional guidance:** Collaborate with healthcare specialists, such as registered dietitians or nutritionists, to create tailored dietary regimens for people with ARFID. Healthcare experts can offer expert advice and help in treating nutritional issues, recognizing nutrient deficiencies, and recommending dietary changes or supplementation as needed.

11

Chapter Eleven

The Power of Mindful Eating

Chapter 12 explores the transformative power of mindful eating in the journey towards healing from Avoidant/Restrictive Food Intake Disorder (ARFID). Mindful eating invites individuals to cultivate a deeper awareness of their eating experiences, reconnect with their senses, and release judgment surrounding food. By embracing mindful eating practices, individuals with ARFID can foster a more nourishing and harmonious relationship with food, supporting their journey towards recovery with compassion and understanding.

Understanding Mindful Eating

Mindful eating is an ancient practice rooted in mindfulness, which involves bringing non-judgmental awareness to the present moment. In the context of eating, mindful eating invites individuals to pay attention to the sensory experience of food, including its taste, texture, smell, and appearance, as well as the thoughts and emotions that arise during eating. Rather than focusing on external rules or restrictions, mindful eating encourages individuals to tune into their internal cues of hunger, fullness, and satisfaction, allowing them to make conscious and intentional choices about what, when, and how much to eat.

Key Principles of Mindful Eating

- **Present Moment Awareness:** Mindful eating involves bringing full attention to the present moment, without judgment or distraction. By cultivating present moment awareness, individuals can fully immerse themselves in the sensory experience of eating, savoring each bite and appreciating the nourishment it provides.
- **Non-Judgmental Observation:** Mindful eating encourages individuals to observe their eating experiences with curiosity and openness, without judging or critiquing themselves. By releasing judgment surrounding food choices, individuals can develop a more compassionate and accepting relationship with food, free from guilt or shame.
- **Savoring the Experience:** Mindful eating invites individuals to savor the experience of eating, paying attention to the flavors, textures, and sensations of each bite. By savoring the experience of eating, individuals can enhance their enjoyment and satisfaction with food, leading to a more positive and fulfilling eating experience.
- **Cultivating Gratitude:** Mindful eating encourages individuals to cultivate gratitude for the food they eat and the nourishment it provides. By appreciating the abundance and variety of foods available to them, individuals can develop a greater sense of connection and appreciation for the role food plays in supporting their health and well-being.
- **Listening to Hunger and Fullness Cues:** Mindful eating involves tuning into internal cues of hunger, fullness, and satisfaction, rather than relying on external rules or restrictions. By listening to their body's signals, individuals can develop a more intuitive and balanced approach to eating, honoring their body's needs and preferences without judgment or criticism.

The Power of Mindful Eating in ARFID Recovery

For individuals with ARFID, mindful eating offers a powerful tool for healing their relationship with food and fostering a sense of empowerment and autonomy in their eating experiences. By embracing mindful eating practices, individuals with ARFID can:

- **Reconnect with Sensory Experiences:** Mindful eating invites individuals to reconnect with the sensory experience of food, allowing them to explore new tastes, textures, and flavors with curiosity and openness. By paying attention to the sensory qualities of food, individuals can develop a greater appreciation for the diversity and richness of the food they eat, leading to a more fulfilling and enjoyable eating experience.

- **Release Judgment and Self-Criticism:** Mindful eating encourages individuals to release judgment and self-criticism surrounding food choices, allowing them to approach eating with compassion and acceptance. By letting go of rigid rules or expectations, individuals can cultivate a more flexible and forgiving attitude towards food, free from guilt or shame.

- **Foster Intuitive Eating:** Mindful eating promotes intuitive eating, which involves listening to internal cues of hunger, fullness, and satisfaction to guide eating behavior. By tuning into their body's signals, individuals with ARFID can develop a greater sense of trust and confidence in their ability to nourish themselves, leading to a more balanced and harmonious relationship with food.

- **Cultivate Mindful Awareness:** Mindful eating cultivates mindful awareness of eating experiences, helping individuals become more attuned to their thoughts, emotions, and sensations surrounding food. By bringing awareness to the present moment, individuals can develop greater insight into their eating behaviors and patterns, empowering them to make conscious and intentional choices about their food intake.

- **Support Emotional Regulation:** Mindful eating can support emotional regulation by helping individuals develop healthier coping strategies for managing stress, anxiety, and other emotional challenges. By cultivating present moment awareness and non-judgmental observation, individuals can learn to respond to emotional triggers with greater resilience and self-compassion, reducing the likelihood of using food as a means of coping with difficult emotions.

Practical Tips for Embracing Mindful Eating

- **Slow Down:** Take time to slow down and savor each bite of food, paying attention to its flavors, textures, and sensations. Avoid rushing through meals or eating on autopilot, and instead, focus on being fully present with the experience of eating.
- **Engage Your Senses:** Engage your senses during meals by noticing the colors, smells, and sounds of the food you eat. Use all your senses to fully immerse yourself in the eating experience, enhancing your enjoyment and satisfaction with food.
- **Practice Gratitude:** Take a moment before eating to express gratitude for the food you are about to enjoy and the nourishment it provides. Cultivate a sense of appreciation for the abundance and variety of foods available to you, fostering a greater connection and appreciation for the role food plays in supporting your health and well-being.
- **Listen to Your Body:** Tune into your body's signals of hunger, fullness, and satisfaction to guide your eating behavior. Pay attention to how different foods make you feel physically and emotionally, and honor your body's needs and preferences without judgment or criticism.
- **Release Judgment:** Let go of judgment and self-criticism surrounding food choices, allowing yourself to eat with compassion and acceptance. Recognize that it's okay to enjoy a wide variety of foods and that there are no "good" or "bad" foods, only choices that nourish and support your well-being.

12

Chapter Twelve

Building Positive Associations with Food

C hapter 12 looks into the transforming practice of developing positive connections with food to overcome Avoidant/Restrictive Food Intake Disorder (ARFID). Individuals with ARFID must form positive associations with food in order to extend their nutritional repertoire, reduce food aversions, and build a healthier relationship with eating. Individuals with ARFID can build confidence, curiosity, and resilience in their journey toward food exploration and recovery by gradually introducing new foods into their diet.

Understanding food aversions in ARFID

Individuals with ARFID frequently have food aversions, which are characterized by extreme anxiety or revulsion towards specific foods or food groups. These aversions are generally caused by sensory sensitivities, poor prior experiences, or underlying anxiety over food. As a result, people with ARFID may restrict their food intake to a small number of "safe" meals, avoiding anything viewed as novel or scary.

The Role of Positive Associations with Food

Building positive associations with food is an important part of ARFID rehabilitation because it helps people overcome their aversions and broaden their dietary options. Individuals with ARFID can establish positive eating experiences by gradually alternating between safe and new meals. This reduces anxiety and increases willingness to try new foods. Positive associations with food include:

- **Reduce Anxiety:** Combining safe and new meals in a supportive and non-threatening atmosphere can help people with ARFID feel more calm and comfortable at mealtimes, lowering anxiety and fear of food.
- **Increase Curiosity:** When people with ARFID have positive experiences with new meals, they may become more interested and open-minded about trying additional foods in the future. Positive food associations can pique people's interest in food exploration, leading to a higher readiness to explore new tastes and sensations.
- **Foster Confidence:** Successfully introducing new foods into meals can enhance people's confidence in their capacity to overcome food-related obstacles and broaden their nutritional repertoire. Building positive associations with food can help people with ARFID feel more confident and self-assured while eating.
- **Build Positive Associations with Food:** Over time, individuals' dietary repertoires might expand as they become more eager to try new foods and flavors. Individuals with ARFID can extend their taste and embrace a more varied and balanced diet by introducing new foods alongside known and preferred items over time.

Strategies for developing positive associations with food:

- **Start tiny:** Begin by combining tiny portions of new meals with familiar and favorite foods that people with ARFID appreciate. Begin with foods that have a similar taste, texture, or appearance to familiar foods, gradually expanding the variety and complexity of new foods over time.

- **Make it Fun:** Make food exploration enjoyable and interactive. Involve people with ARFID in meal planning, grocery shopping, and food preparation activities, allowing them to take control of their food choices and develop a sense of joy and anticipation about trying new things.

- **Offer awards and Reinforcement:** Provide awards and positive reinforcement to people with ARFID for their efforts in trying new foods, regardless of the results. Celebrate little victories and successes along the way to reinforce positive connections with food and encourage future exploration and experimentation.

- **Be Patient and Supportive:**Be patient and supportive as people with ARFID manage their food exploration adventure. Encourage children to try new meals with an open mind, free of pressure or judgement. Offer reassurance and support, recognizing their bravery and efforts to venture outside of their comfort zone.

- **Model Healthy Eating Behaviours:** Be a positive role model for those with ARFID by showing healthy eating habits and attitudes. Share your personal experiences with trying new foods and show your passion and enjoyment of eating, enabling those with ARFID to approach food discovery with confidence and optimism.

Case Study: Sarah's Journey Towards Building Positive Associations with Food.

Sarah, a 10-year-old girl diagnosed with ARFID, eats mostly chicken nuggets, French fries, and plain pasta. Despite her parents' efforts to introduce new cuisines, Sarah is hesitant and nervous about trying anything new. Sarah starts on a journey towards developing positive connections with food, with the help of a licensed dietician and therapist.

Gradual Exposure: Sarah's therapist assists her in developing a hierarchy of fearful foods, beginning with those that are similar in taste or texture to her safe foods. They start with tiny servings of mashed potatoes and her favorite chicken nuggets, gradually increasing the variety and complexity of new foods over time.

Fun and Interactive Approach: Sarah's parents involve her in meal planning and preparation activities, giving her the opportunity to taste new foods and experiment with different recipes and flavors. They make food exploration exciting and participatory by turning mealtime into a game, utilizing colorful plates and cutlery, and integrating themed dinners based on other cuisines.

Positive Reinforcement: Sarah's parents provide rewards and positive re-inforcement for her efforts to try new meals, such as stickers or little gifts. They applaud her boldness and desire to move outside of her comfort zone, reinforcing positive connections with food and encouraging more exploration.

Patience and Support: Sarah's therapist and dietician provide continual support and encouragement as she embarks on her food exploration journey. They affirm her feelings and experiences, recognizing the difficulties she faces and assuring her that it is acceptable to take tiny steps toward tasting new foods.

Modeling Healthy Eating Behaviours: Sarah's parents model healthy eating habits and attitudes by being enthusiastic about trying new foods. They tell Sarah about their own food exploration experiences and convey their joy and curiosity about experiencing new flavors and cuisines, inspiring her to approach food with a spirit of adventure and openness.

13

Chapter Thirteen

Celebrating Progress and Managing Setbacks

Chapter 13 discusses the importance of celebrating progress and dealing with setbacks on the path to recovery from Avoidant/Restrictive Food Intake Disorder (ARFID). Recovery from ARFID is a difficult and complex process marked by both successes and failures. Individuals with ARFID can stay motivated and move on with courage and drive on their route to recovery by embracing progress, learning from failures, and fostering resilience.

Celebrate Progress

Celebrating success is an important component of ARFID recovery because it recognizes individuals' efforts and achievements as they try to extend their dietary repertoire and overcome food aversions. Celebrating achievement enables people to recognize their strengths, gain confidence, and stay motivated on their path to healing. Some important ways to recognize success in ARFID rehabilitation include:

- **Recognize Small successes:** Celebrate even the tiniest successes and accomplishments in ARFID recovery, such as trying new food, broadening the range of safe foods, or eating without worry or discomfort. Recognize the courage and effort required for people with ARFID to move out of their comfort zone and try new things.

- **Set Milestones and Goals:** Set precise objectives and targets for ARFID recovery, and celebrate each step along the way. Setting attainable goals, whether it's trying a new food every week, widening the spectrum of safe foods, or effectively navigating a difficult eating circumstance, gives people a feeling of direction and progress in their recovery.

- **Express gratitude:** Express gratitude to family, friends, therapists, and other members of your support network for their help and encouragement. Take the time to acknowledge the importance that others play in ARFID recovery and show your gratitude for their continued support and encouragement.

- **Reflect on Progress:** Take time to consider the progress made in ARFID recovery, noting the challenges conquered, lessons learned, and personal growth that occurred along the road. Reflecting on progress can help people recognize their tenacity and determination in the face of hardship, giving them a sense of pride and success.

- **Celebrate Self-Care:** In ARFID recovery, recognize the significance of prioritizing one's physical, emotional, and mental well-being. Whether it's relaxing, participating in fun activities, or practicing mindfulness, celebrating self-care emphasizes the significance of supporting oneself during the healing process.

Managing setbacks

While recognizing success is crucial, it is also critical to recognize and navigate setbacks that may arise throughout ARFID recovery. Setbacks are a normal aspect of the healing process and offer opportunities for learning, growth, and resilience. Individuals with ARFID can overcome barriers and continue their recovery journey by taking a proactive and compassionate attitude to dealing with setbacks. Here are some critical ideas for addressing setbacks in ARFID recovery:

- **Normalise Setbacks:** Understand that setbacks are a typical and expected part of the ARFID rehabilitation process. Instead of perceiving setbacks as failures, consider them opportunities for learning and progress. Normalise setbacks as transient setbacks on the road to long-term healing and recovery.
- **Identify Triggers and Patterns:** Determine the factors and patterns that contribute to setbacks in ARFID recovery, such as stressful events, routine changes, or unpleasant emotions. Understanding the fundamental causes of setbacks allows individuals to build strategies for managing and limiting their impact in the future.
- **Practice Self-Compassion:** When dealing with obstacles in ARFID rehabilitation, practice self-compassion and gentleness towards oneself. Be kind and forgiving to yourself, remembering that setbacks are a normal part of the healing process and do not determine your worth or progress. Treat yourself with the same compassion and understanding that you would show a friend facing comparable circumstances.
- **Seek Support:** When faced with obstacles in ARFID recovery, seek help from family, friends, therapists, and other members of your support network. Share your feelings openly and honestly, and seek advice and support from those who understand and empathize with your difficulties. Remember that you are not alone on your trip, and individuals are willing to help you every step of the way.
- **Learn from Setbacks:** Consider setbacks as chances for learning and growth in ARFID rehabilitation. Consider the elements that contributed to the setback, identify any patterns or triggers, and devise ways to avoid similar setbacks in the future. Setbacks can serve as excellent learning experiences, informing and strengthening your approach to recovery in the future.

Case Study: James' Journey of Celebrating Progress and Navigating Setbacks

James, a 25-year-old man diagnosed with ARFID, has been working hard with a therapist and qualified dietitian to broaden his dietary options and conquer his food aversions. Over the last three months, James has made considerable strides in tasting new meals and addressing his avoidance behaviors. He has successfully added various new fruits and vegetables to his diet and has even experimented with new recipes at home.

Despite his improvement, James faces a setback when he attends a social gathering where unusual dishes are presented. James, feeling overwhelmed and uncomfortable, reverts to familiar, safe foods while shunning new dishes entirely. James is frustrated and doubts himself because he is unable to overcome his food aversions at present.

In the days following the social gathering, James reflects on the setback and seeks support from his therapist. Together, they investigate the factors and feelings that contributed to the setback, such as social anxiety and fear of judgment. James learns that setbacks are a normal part of the healing process and do not negate the progress he has achieved thus far.

James works with his therapist to establish future methods for controlling social anxiety and negotiating difficult eating circumstances. He uses relaxation techniques like deep breathing and visualization to help calm his anxiety and stay anchored in the moment. James also turns to friends and family for help, openly expressing his experiences and seeking encouragement from individuals who understand and support his recovery process.

As James continues to reflect on the setback and practice coping skills, he gains a new sense of enthusiasm and resolve in his ARFID recovery. He understands that setbacks are chances for learning and growth, and he is determined to use this experience to build his resilience and accelerate his progress towards conquering his food aversions.

14

Chapter 14

Long-Term Management and Maintaining Recovery

Chapter 14 focuses on long-term treatment and rehabilitation from Avoidant/Restrictive Food Intake Disorder (ARFID). While making initial progress in ARFID recovery is a big step forward, long-term recovery takes continual dedication, perseverance, and support. Individuals with ARFID can manage the challenges of daily living with confidence and resilience by employing relapse prevention measures and taking a long-term approach to recovery.

Understanding Long-Term Management for ARFID Recovery:

Long-term management in ARFID recovery entails adopting methods and behaviors that promote ongoing development, resilience, and well-being beyond the initial stages of therapy. It includes a variety of self-care strategies, coping skills, and lifestyle changes aimed at maintaining a healthy and rewarding relationship with food and eating. Long-term management for ARFID recovery focuses on:

· **Relapse Prevention:** Preventing relapse is an important part of long-term management in ARFID recovery, as setbacks and problems can occur even after significant improvement is made. Relapse prevention tactics assist individuals in identifying triggers, developing coping skills, and navigating potential obstacles in order to sustain their recovery and prevent the recurrence of disordered eating behaviors.

- **Sustainable Practices:** Implementing sustainable practices enhances consistency and stability in ARFID recovery, allowing individuals to retain their success over time. Sustainable practices include good eating habits, self-care routines, and coping skills that may be incorporated into everyday life and modified to meet changing circumstances.
- **Building Resilience:** Building resilience is critical for long-term management in ARFID recovery because it allows people to recover from setbacks, deal with stress, and face difficulties with strength and resolve. Building resilience entails learning coping skills, forming social support networks, and establishing a positive mentality that encourages flexibility and perseverance.
- **Self-Compassion and Acceptance:** Self-compassion and acceptance are essential for long-term management in ARFID recovery because they promote a gentle and nonjudgmental attitude towards oneself and one's experiences. Self-compassion and acceptance assist people to develop self-esteem, self-worth, and self-acceptance, which promotes resilience and well-being in the face of hardship.
- **Continued Growth and Learning:** Adopting a growth mindset and committing to lifelong learning is critical for long-term success in ARFID recovery. Seeking opportunities for personal and professional development, exploring new interests and hobbies, and forcing oneself to step beyond of one's comfort zone and accept new experiences all contribute to ongoing growth and learning.

Relapse Prevention Strategies

Relapse prevention tactics are proactive measures that try to identify and mitigate potential triggers and risk factors for relapse in ARFID treatment. These tactics assist individuals in anticipating and responding to problems successfully, lowering the risk of setbacks while fostering long-term progress and well-being. Some important relapse prevention measures in ARFID rehabilitation include:

- **Identify Triggers:** Determine potential relapse triggers, such as stressful situations, changes in habit, or unpleasant feelings. Recognizing triggers allows individuals to build effective ways of managing them and lowering their impact on eating behaviors.

- **Develop Coping Skills:** Learn how to handle triggers and negotiate difficult situations without succumbing to disordered eating behaviors. Relaxation techniques, problem-solving strategies, assertiveness training, and mindfulness practices can all be used as coping tools.

- **Create a supportive environment:** Surround oneself with a caring environment that encourages recovery and well-being. Develop relationships with friends, family members, therapists, and support groups that understand and empathize with your experiences and can offer encouragement, advice, and reassurance.

- **Establish Healthy Routines:** Create healthy routines and habits that promote physical, emotional, and mental well-being. Prioritize regular meals and snacks, enough sleep, physical activity, stress management, and self-care activities that promote balance and resilience in your daily life.

- **Monitor Progress:** Check in on your ARFID recovery on a frequent basis to track changes, detect patterns, and recognize symptoms of potential relapse. Keep a notebook or diary to record your thoughts, feelings, and behaviors about food and eating, and use this information to find areas for improvement and change.

A Sustainable Approach to Recovery

A sustainable approach to recovery in ARFID entails implementing strategies and behaviors that promote long-term well-being and resilience while respecting individual needs, preferences, and values. A long-term approach to rehabilitation emphasizes flexibility, self-compassion, and balance, enabling people to negotiate life's ups and downs with grace and resilience. Some critical components of a sustainable approach to rehabilitation in ARFID are:

- **Flexible Eating Habits:** Develop eating habits that allow for individual tastes, nutritional demands, and lifestyle considerations. Incorporate a variety of foods into your meals and snacks, but also allow for occasional indulgences and delights without feeling guilty or judged.
- **Self-care Practices:** Prioritise self-care techniques that promote physical, emotional, and mental well. Meditation, yoga, deep breathing exercises, writing, and spending time in nature are all good ways to relax, relieve stress, and regulate emotions.
- **Balanced Lifestyle:** Strive for balance in all aspects of your life, including work, relationships, leisure, and personal care. Create a balanced lifestyle that includes rest, recreation, social interaction, personal development, and meaningful activities that offer you joy and fulfillment.
- **Cultivate Social Support:** Build a strong network of friends, family members, therapists, and support groups who understand and encourage your recovery. During difficult times, rely on your support network for encouragement, guidance, and reassurance, and return the favor by helping others.
- **Self-Compassion:** Practice self-compassion and acceptance of oneself and one's experiences during ARFID rehabilitation. Be patient and forgiving with yourself, understanding that development is not always linear and that setbacks are a normal part of the healing process. Treat yourself with care, tolerance, and patience, and acknowledge your accomplishments along the road.

Case Study: Emma's Journey to Long-Term Management and Recovery

Emma, a 30-year-old woman diagnosed with ARFID, has been on the road to recovery for several years. Emma's therapist, certified dietitian, and support network have helped her extend her dietary range, challenge her food aversions, and build healthier eating habits.

Emma faces several hurdles and setbacks in her recovery road. Despite these obstacles, Emma remains devoted to her recovery and uses relapse prevention tactics and long-term practices to maintain her success and well-being.

Emma identifies her relapse triggers, such as intense job deadlines and social gatherings with unfamiliar meals, and develops coping strategies to effectively handle them. She uses relaxation techniques like deep breathing and visualization to soothe her nerves and lessen anxiety in stressful times. Emma also sets healthy habits, such as regular meal times, enough sleep, and daily self-care activities, to support her physical, emotional, and mental well-being.

In addition to relapse prevention measures, Emma takes a long-term approach to recovery that emphasizes flexibility, balance, and self-compassion. She cultivates adaptable eating habits that allow for a wide range of foods and occasional indulgences without guilt or judgment. Emma prioritizes self-care methods that encourage relaxation, stress alleviation, and emotional regulation, such as nature walks, yoga, and journaling.

Emma also builds a solid support network of friends, family members, and recovery peers who understand and empathize with her difficulties. During difficult times, she relies on her support network for encouragement, guidance, and reassurance, and she returns the favor by helping others.

Emma is making progress in her path to healing from ARFID thanks to her dedication to long-term management and rehabilitation. She believes in relapse prevention tactics and long-term practices that foster resilience, well-being, and self-compassion, helping her to face life's ups and downs with grace and resolve.

IV

Part 4: ARFID in Adults and Children

15

Chapter Fifteen

ARFID in Children

Chapter 16 provides particular techniques for parents and carers of children with Avoidant/Restrictive Food Intake Disorder (ARFID). Navigating ARFID in children can be difficult, but with the correct aid, communication, and methods, parents and carers can help their children overcome food aversions, broaden their nutritional repertoire, and thrive in their relationship with food.

Understanding ARFID in children

ARFID in children is defined by selective or limited eating behaviors, avoidance of specific foods or food groups, and severe distress or impairment associated with eating. Children with ARFID may have sensory sensitivity, a fear of choking or vomiting, or other underlying disorders that impede their eating abilities. Parents and carers must recognize that ARFID is a serious eating disorder that requires support, awareness, and action.

Communication Strategies for Parents and Carers

Effective communication is essential for aiding children with ARFID and overcoming their food aversions. Here are some communication suggestions for parents and carers:

- **Create a Safe and Supportive Environment:** Make sure that children feel comfortable sharing their thoughts, feelings, and worries regarding food and eating. Instead of putting pressure or judgment on children, show them empathy, compassion, and support.
- **Listen Actively:** Actively listen to children's concerns and eating experiences. Validate their emotions and recognize the difficulties they experience, displaying empathy and understanding.
- **Encourage Open Dialogue:** Encourage open discussion about food and eating, allowing children to voice their likes, dislikes, and preferences without fear of being judged or criticized. Encourage a collaborative approach to meal planning and preparation, including children in decision-making and giving them a say in their food choices.
- **Provide Reassurance and Support:** Assist children in navigating their food aversions and eating issues. Remind them that it is acceptable to take baby steps towards tasting new foods and that progress requires time and patience.
- **Model Healthy Eating Behaviours:** Be a positive role model for children by displaying healthy eating habits and attitudes. Share your personal experiences with tasting new foods and communicate your excitement and delight in eating, encouraging children to approach food with curiosity and openness.
- **Seek Professional Help:** Consult pediatricians, qualified dietitians, therapists, and other healthcare providers who specialize in treating ARFID in children. Work with healthcare professionals to create a thorough treatment plan that is personalized to your child's unique needs and preferences.

Navigating School Meals

Children with ARFID have additional obstacles at school meals, such as unfamiliar foods, social pressure, and limited selections. Here are some ways to manage school meals:

- **Communicate with School Staff:** Inform teachers, administrators, and cafeteria workers about your child's nutritional needs and preferences. Provide information regarding ARFID and any particular accommodations or modifications that may be required to meet your child's needs.
- **Pack Familiar Foods:** Include familiar and favored foods from home that your child enjoys and is comfortable eating. Include a variety of nutritional options, such as fruits and vegetables, whole grains, and protein sources, to ensure that your child's meals and snacks are balanced and satisfying throughout the school day.
- **Provide Encouragement and Support:** Encourage and support your child as they navigates school meals. Provide reassurance that it is acceptable to bring their food from home and that they can eat whatever feels secure and comfortable to them.
- **Educate classmates and Teachers:** Inform your child's classmates and teachers about ARFID and how they may assist your child during mealtimes. Encourage students to be understanding and inclusive, and give teachers information and ideas for fostering a friendly and inclusive lunch atmosphere.
- **Collaborate with School Professionals:** Work with school counselors, nurses, and psychologists to create a support plan for your child's ARFID in school. Work together to identify triggers, make accommodations, and provide emotional support so that your child feels safe and supported at mealtimes.

More Strategies for Parents and Carers

In addition to communication suggestions and techniques for negotiating school meals, here are some further strategies for parents and carers of children with ARFID:

- **Seek Professional Help:** Consult pediatricians, qualified dietitians, therapists, and other healthcare providers who specialize in treating ARFID in children. Work with healthcare professionals to create a thorough treatment plan that is personalized to your child's unique needs and preferences.
- **Provide structure and routine:** Provide structure and regularity around mealtimes to ensure that your child has a predictable and supportive dining setting. Set regular meal and snack times, provide a range of nutritional alternatives, and limit distractions to help your youngster concentrate on eating.
- **Offer Choices and Autonomy:** Allow your youngster to choose what and how much to eat during mealtimes. Respect your child's tastes and avoid pressuring them to consume items they dislike.
- **Celebrate Progress:** Recognise your child's ARFID recovery progress and successes, no matter how minor. Recognize their bravery and efforts in trying new foods, extending their dietary palette, and confronting their concerns with courage and drive.
- **Self-Care:** As a parent or carer, you should prioritize your own physical, emotional, and mental well. Make time for relaxation, hobbies, and activities that offer you joy and fulfillment, and seek assistance from friends, family, and support groups as needed.

16

Chapter Sixteen

ARFID in Adults

Chapter 17 delves into the unique challenges and considerations experienced by adults with Avoidant/Restrictive Food Intake Disorder (ARFID). While ARFID is commonly associated with children and teenagers, it can remain into adulthood, posing unique issues in social interactions, connections with food, and overall well-being.

Understanding ARFID in Adults

ARFID in adults is distinguished by selective or limited eating behaviors, avoidance of specific foods or food groups, and severe distress or impairment associated with eating. Adults with ARFID may have long-standing food aversions, sensory sensitivities, or other underlying disorders that affect their eating habits. ARFID, unlike other eating disorders, is motivated by food-related fear, anxiety, or discomfort rather than body image concerns or weight loss goals.

Unique Challenges Faced by Adults with ARFID

Adults with ARFID encounter a wide range of particular issues and considerations that affect their everyday lives and overall well-being. Some of these challenges are:

- **Social Situations:** Adults with ARFID may experience pressure to eat novel foods or negotiate social expectations surrounding meals and dining out. Attending social gatherings, parties, or business functions that entail food can cause anxiety and discomfort, resulting in avoidance or withdrawal from social engagements.

- **Relationships with Food:** Adults with ARFID may struggle with their connection with food, experiencing dread, anxiety, or guilt when eating or at mealtimes. They may have strict dietary preferences or routines, dislike certain textures or flavors, or suffer from sensory sensitivities that make eating difficult or unpleasant. These issues can have an influence on their nutritional intake, physical health, and general quality of life.

- **Mental Health and Well-being:** Living with ARFID can hurt an adult's mental health and well-being, including feelings of loneliness, frustration, and low self-esteem. They may feel anxiety, depression, or other mental health issues as a result of their eating problems and the consequences for their social, personal, and professional lives. Seeking help from mental health specialists and engaging in self-care routines are critical for emotional resilience and well-being.

- **Seeking Treatment and Support:** Adults with ARFID may experience obstacles to receiving treatment and support, including a lack of information about the disease, the stigma associated with mental health issues, or difficulty accessing specialized care. Finding educated healthcare practitioners, therapists, and support groups who understand ARFID and can give successful therapy and support is critical to adult recovery and well-being.

Strategies for Using ARFID as an Adult

Regardless of the problems they endure, adults with ARFID can negotiate their experiences with perseverance, self-compassion, and successful eating techniques. Here are some tips for navigating ARFID as an adult:

- **Advocate for Yourself:** Speak up for yourself and your needs in social interactions, relationships, and healthcare settings. Be forceful in communicating your food and eating choices, boundaries, and concerns, and seek concessions or modifications that promote your health and comfort.
- **Practice Self-Compassion:** As you manage the challenges of living with ARFID, be gentle to yourself. Recognize the strength and grit required to face your concerns, try new meals, and seek help for your eating issues. Treat yourself with the same compassion and understanding that you would show a friend facing comparable circumstances.
- **Develop coping strategies:** Create coping techniques for dealing with anxiety, discomfort, or triggers associated with food and eating. Deep breathing, mindfulness, and progressive muscle relaxation are all relaxation techniques that can help you calm down and minimize stress during meals or social situations. Engage in activities that provide you joy and relaxation, such as spending time outside, listening to music, or doing something you enjoy.
- **Seek Support:** Talk to friends, family members, and support groups who understand and empathize with your ARFID experiences. Share your struggles, worries, and triumphs with your support network, and seek encouragement, validation, and reassurance. Consider joining online communities or support groups for people with ARFID to connect with others who have had similar experiences and can provide mutual support and understanding.
- **Engage in Treatment:** Seek help for ARFID from educated healthcare experts, therapists, and registered dietitians who specialize in eating disorders. Investigate therapeutic approaches such as cognitive-behavioral therapy (CBT), exposure therapy, or acceptance and commitment therapy

(ACT), which address the underlying causes of your eating difficulties and offer strategies for managing symptoms and improving your relationship with food.

- **Set Realistic Goals:** As you embark on your ARFID recovery path, set realistic and achievable goals for yourself. Break down huge goals into smaller, more doable steps, and celebrate each milestone and achievement along the way. Recognize that development may be sluggish and nonlinear, and be patient and compassionate with yourself as you strive for your goals.

Case Study: Alex's Experience With ARFID as an Adult

Alex, a 35-year-old man, has struggled with ARFID since childhood, causing anxiety and discomfort around specific foods and textures. As an adult, Alex finds distinct problems in handling his eating difficulties while leading a full and balanced life:

Social circumstances: Alex feels anxious and uncomfortable in social circumstances involving food, and he frequently avoids parties or occasions where strange meals will be served. He feels alone and lonely and wishes he could participate more fully in social events without fear of being judged or scrutinized.

Relationships with Food: Alex's connection with food is exacerbated by his ARFID, which causes him to feel fear, anxiety, and guilt when he eats or has a meal. He avoids different textures and flavors in favor of familiar foods that make him feel safe and comfortable, resulting in nutritional deficits and physical health difficulties.

Mental Health and Well-being: Living with ARFID hurts Alex's mental health and well-being, causing him to experience irritation, low self-esteem, and sadness as a result of his eating troubles. He receives help from an eating disorder therapist, who works with him to identify the underlying causes of his ARFID and build coping methods to manage his symptoms.

Seeking Treatment and Support: Alex experiences difficulties in obtaining specialized treatment and support for his ARFID since he struggles to find healthcare experts who understand and have experience treating adults with the illness. He advocates for himself and educates his healthcare professionals about ARFID, requesting referrals to specialists and support organizations who can give successful therapy and support during his rehabilitation.

17

Conclusion

Managing Avoidant/Restrictive Food Intake Disorder (ARFID) poses distinct problems and considerations, whether in children or adults. Throughout this book, we've looked at a variety of methods, insights, and coping mechanisms designed for different stages and features of ARFID recovery.

From understanding the causes of ARFID to embracing long-term management and relapse prevention, we've delved into the nuances of this illness, providing practical advice and support. We've emphasized the value of communication, self-compassion, and seeking expert assistance, emphasizing the strength and commitment required to overcome ARFID's challenges.

Whether you're a parent supporting a child with ARFID or an adult navigating your journey, remember that you're not alone. By promoting empathy, understanding, and collaboration, we can build a community in which people with ARFID feel heard, supported, and empowered to live their lives to the fullest.

As you continue your journey to healing and well-being, remember to celebrate every step forward, no matter how tiny. Each difficulty is overcome, fear tackled, and each moment of growth demonstrates your strength and courage.